DIABETIC PCOS DIET COOKBOOK

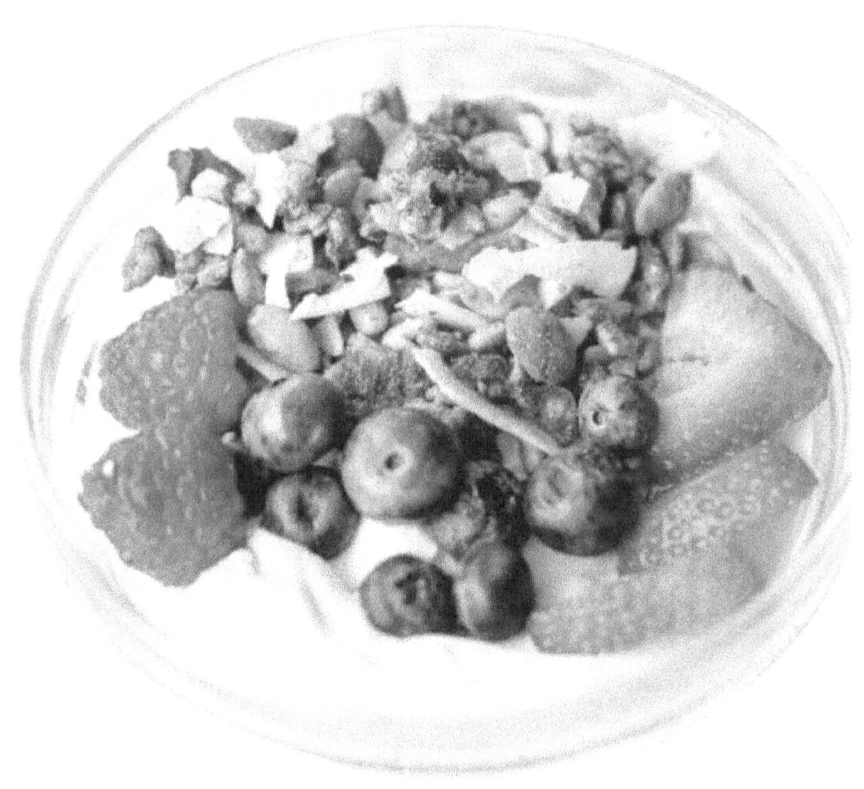

LYSANDRA QUINN

DISCLAIMER

The content within this book reflects my thoughts, experiences, and beliefs. It is meant for informational and entertainment purposes. While I have taken great care to provide accurate information, I cannot guarantee the absolute correctness or applicability of the content to every individual or situation. Please consult with relevant professionals for advice specific to your needs.

Contact the Author

Thank you for reading my book! I would love to hear from you, whether you have feedback, questions, or just want to share your thoughts. Your feedback means a lot to me and helps me improve as a writer.

Please don't hesitate to reach out to me through

contactmelysandraquinn@gmail.com

I look forward to connecting with my readers and appreciate your support in this literary journey. Your thoughts and comments are valuable to me.

TABLE OF CONTENTS

INTRODUCTION

In the quiet corners of our lives, where challenges loom large and hope seems elusive, sometimes it takes the simplest of recipes to weave magic into our existence. This is a tale that begins with a friend, Sophie, whose journey through the maze of PCOS and diabetes echoed the struggles of countless women around the world. A tale of resilience, triumph, and the transformative power of a carefully curated PCOS diet.

It was a chilly evening when Sophie, with a weary smile on her face, confided in me about her relentless battle with PCOS and diabetes. Having scoured through a plethora of cookbooks, each promising a miraculous solution, she found herself trapped in a cycle of disappointment. Countless recipes later, she stood on the precipice of surrender, until a glimmer of hope emerged.

As a seasoned dietician with over two decades of experience, my journey into the intricate world of PCOS recipes was not one born out of mere curiosity, but rather out of a sense of duty to help those like Sophie. The countless hours of research, trials, and fine-tuning were motivated by a singular desire: to create a collection of recipes that could offer relief where others had fallen short.

For years, I had observed the impact of various dietary approaches on PCOS, dissecting the nuances, understanding the intricate dance between nutrition and hormones. When Sophie approached me with a plea for guidance, I felt compelled to share my culinary arsenal – a compilation of recipes that had evolved over years of careful crafting.

The transformation in Sophie's life was nothing short of remarkable. Gone were the days of fluctuating energy levels, mood swings, and the daunting challenge of managing diabetes alongside PCOS. The recipes worked in harmony to bring balance to her life, igniting a spark of hope that had long been extinguished.

The decision to pen down these recipes was not a mere professional endeavor but a heartfelt response to the silent cries of women struggling with similar afflictions. As a dietician, I've witnessed the profound impact that food can have on the body and mind. This cookbook is not just a collection of recipes; it's a lifeline for those seeking a path to wellness.

Now, as I present this cookbook to you, dear reader, I implore you to reflect on the challenges you or your loved ones face. Can a single meal change the course of your health journey? Can a cookbook be more than just a compilation of recipes, but a companion in your pursuit of a healthier, happier life?

Imagine waking up each morning with a renewed sense of energy, bidding farewell to the days of uncertainty and embracing a life where food is not just sustenance but a powerful ally in your fight against PCOS and diabetes. Picture a dining table adorned with delicious dishes that not only tantalize your taste buds but also nourish your body from within.

As you embark on this culinary journey, allow yourself to be guided by the stories of transformation woven into each recipe. What if, within these pages, lies the key to unlocking a life free from the shackles of PCOS and diabetes? Can you afford to let this opportunity slip through your fingers?

This cookbook is more than a compilation of recipes; it's a testament to the transformative power of nutrition. It's a whisper of encouragement for those navigating the challenging terrain of PCOS and diabetes. Join me in embracing the magic that lies within these pages, and let each bite bring you closer to the harmonious life you deserve.

CHAPTER 1

THE BASICS OF PCOS AND DIABETES

Polycystic Ovary Syndrome, commonly known as PCOS, is a hormonal disorder that affects individuals with ovaries, typically during their reproductive years. This condition is characterized by the overproduction of androgens, which are male hormones, and the presence of small fluid-filled sacs (cysts) on the ovaries. PCOS can lead to various symptoms, including irregular menstrual cycles, ovulatory dysfunction, acne, excessive hair growth (hirsutism), and weight gain. It is also associated with an increased risk of developing other health conditions, including diabetes.

Understanding Diabetes:

Diabetes is a chronic medical condition that occurs when the body is unable to properly regulate blood sugar (glucose) levels. There are two main types of diabetes: Type 1 diabetes, which is an autoimmune condition where the body does not produce insulin, and Type 2 diabetes, which is characterized by insulin resistance, where the body's cells do not respond effectively to insulin.

Insulin is a hormone produced by the pancreas that helps regulate blood sugar levels. When there is a deficiency of insulin or the body's cells do not respond adequately to it, blood sugar levels can become elevated, leading to various health complications. Diabetes can result in symptoms such as increased thirst, frequent urination, fatigue, and slow wound healing.

The Link between PCOS and Diabetes:

There is a significant association between PCOS and diabetes, particularly Type 2 diabetes. Women with PCOS are at an increased risk of developing insulin resistance, which is a key factor in the development of Type 2 diabetes. Insulin resistance occurs when the body's cells do not respond efficiently to insulin, causing an elevated level of glucose in the bloodstream.

In PCOS, the hormonal imbalances, including elevated levels of androgens, can contribute to insulin resistance. Additionally, obesity, which is common in individuals with PCOS, further exacerbates insulin resistance. Insulin resistance can lead to higher levels of insulin in the body, which, over time, can contribute to the development of Type 2 diabetes.

Managing PCOS and Diabetes:

For individuals with PCOS, managing the condition involves addressing both the hormonal imbalances and the associated risks, including the risk of diabetes. Lifestyle modifications, such as a healthy diet, regular exercise, and weight management, play a crucial role in improving insulin sensitivity and reducing the risk of diabetes. In some cases, medications such as oral contraceptives or insulin-sensitizing agents may be prescribed to help regulate hormonal levels and manage symptoms.

Regular monitoring of blood sugar levels and adopting a proactive approach to overall health are essential for individuals with PCOS to reduce the risk of developing diabetes and its associated complications. Collaboration between healthcare providers, including gynecologists and endocrinologists, is often necessary to provide comprehensive care for individuals with PCOS and diabetes.

CHAPTER 2

BUILDING A BALANCED PCOS AND DIABETES-FRIENDLY PLATE

When managing both Polycystic Ovary Syndrome (PCOS) and diabetes, creating a balanced and nutritious plate is crucial for maintaining stable blood sugar levels and promoting overall health. Here's a guide on how to structure your meals for optimal management of these conditions.

Macronutrient Breakdown: Carbohydrates, Proteins, Fats:

Carbohydrates:

Choose complex carbohydrates with a low glycemic index (GI), such as whole grains, legumes, and vegetables. These foods release glucose into the bloodstream more gradually, preventing rapid spikes in blood sugar.

Monitor portion sizes to control carbohydrate intake and distribute them evenly throughout the day.

Proteins:

Incorporate lean proteins like poultry, fish, tofu, legumes, and low-fat dairy into your meals. Protein helps stabilize blood sugar levels and promotes satiety.

Include a source of protein in each meal to support muscle health and regulate hunger.

Fats:

Opt for healthy fats, including avocados, nuts, seeds, and olive oil. These fats have cardiovascular benefits and can contribute to better insulin sensitivity.

Be mindful of portion sizes, as fats are energy dense. Focus on unsaturated fats and limit saturated and trans fats.

Portion Control for Blood Sugar Management:

Balanced Portions:

Divide your plate into sections for carbohydrates, proteins, and vegetables. This method ensures a balanced intake of nutrients.

Aim for smaller, frequent meals throughout the day to prevent large spikes in blood sugar.

Monitoring Carbohydrate Portions:

Pay attention to carbohydrate servings, considering the impact on blood sugar. Use measuring tools or visual cues to estimate appropriate portions.

Include a variety of colorful vegetables, which are rich in fiber and essential nutrients.

Protein Portion Management:

Opt for appropriate protein portions based on your individual needs. This can help stabilize blood sugar and promote feelings of fullness.

Experiment with different protein sources to add variety to your meals.

Healthy Fats in Moderation:

While healthy fats are beneficial, moderate your portions. Use small amounts of olive oil, nuts, or avocados to enhance flavor and satiety.

Avoid fried and heavily processed foods high in unhealthy fats.

Creating Balanced Meals:

Include a Variety of Foods:

Diversify your diet with a range of nutrient-dense foods to ensure you get a broad spectrum of vitamins and minerals.

Rotate protein sources, grains, and vegetables to prevent monotony.

Mindful Eating:

Practice mindful eating by savoring each bite, chewing slowly, and paying attention to hunger and fullness cues.

Minimize distractions during meals to foster a better connection with your body's signals.

Hydration:

Stay adequately hydrated with water or herbal teas. Limit sugary beverages, as they can contribute to blood sugar spikes.

Consider spreading water intake throughout the day.

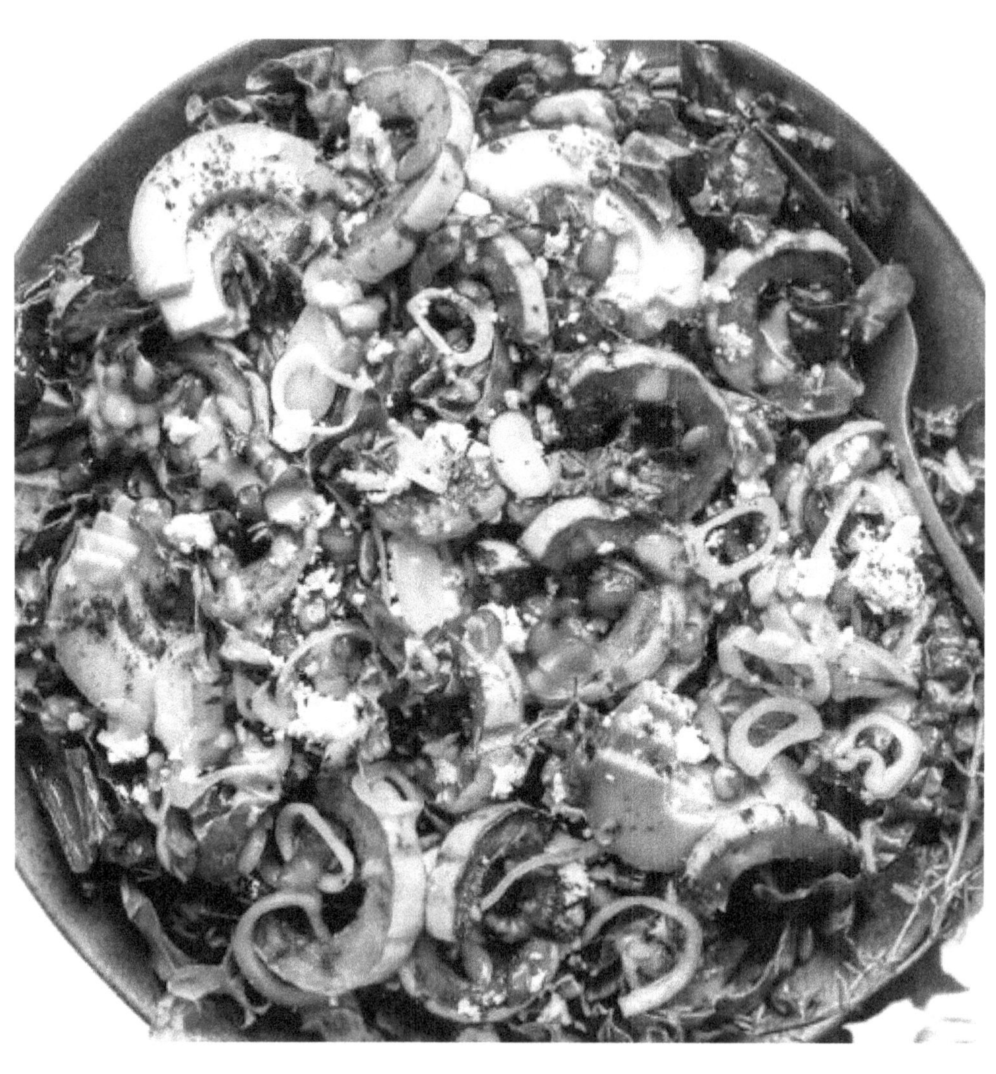

CHAPTER 3

PCOS AND DIABETES-FRIENDLY

BREAKFAST RECIPES

Vegetable Omelets with Whole Grain Toast:

Cooking Time: 15 minutes

Serving: 1

Ingredients:

- 2 eggs
- Assorted vegetables (bell peppers, spinach, tomatoes)
- 1 slice of whole grain bread

Instructions:

1. Whisk eggs and pour into a heated, non-stick pan.
2. Add chopped vegetables to the eggs and cook until set.
3. Toast the whole grain bread.
4. Serve the vegetable omelet on the toast.

Nutritional Information:

Calories: 300, Carbs: 25g, Protein: 20g, Fat: 12g, Fiber: 5g

Greek Yogurt Parfait with Berries and Almonds:

Cooking Time: 5 minutes

Serving: 1

Ingredients:

- 1 cup Greek yogurt
- Mixed berries (strawberries, blueberries)
- 1 tablespoon almonds (chopped)

Instructions:

1. Layer Greek yogurt with mixed berries in a glass or bowl.
2. Top with chopped almonds.
3. Repeat layers for a visually appealing parfait.

Nutritional Information:

Calories: 250, Carbs: 30g, Protein: 20g, Fat: 8g, Fiber: 6g

Quinoa Breakfast Bowl with Nuts and Cinnamon:

Cooking Time: 20 minutes

Serving: 1

Ingredients:

- 1/2 cup cooked quinoa
- 1/4 cup mixed nuts (almonds, walnuts)
- Dash of cinnamon
- 1 tablespoon honey (optional)

Instructions:

1. Cook quinoa according to package instructions.
2. Mix in mixed nuts and sprinkle with cinnamon.
3. Drizzle with honey if desired.

Nutritional Information:

Calories: 320, Carbs: 40g, Protein: 10g, Fat: 15g, Fiber: 5g

Chia Seed Pudding with Coconut and Mango:

Preparation Time: 5 minutes (plus overnight refrigeration)

Serving: 1

Ingredients:

- 2 tablespoons chia seeds
- 1/2 cup unsweetened almond milk
- 1/4 cup diced mango.
- 1 tablespoon shredded coconut

Instructions:

1. Mix chia seeds and almond milk; refrigerate overnight.
2. In the morning, layer chia pudding with diced mango and shredded coconut.

Nutritional Information:

Calories: 280, Carbs: 30g, Protein: 7g, Fat: 15g, Fiber: 10g

Whole Grain Pancakes with Greek Yogurt and Berries:

Cooking Time: 20 minutes

Serving: 2

Ingredients:

- 1 cup whole grain pancake mix
- 1 cup water
- 1 cup Greek yogurt
- Mixed berries for topping

Instructions:

1. Prepare pancake batter with water.
2. Cook pancakes on a griddle.
3. Top with a dollop of Greek yogurt and mixed berries.

Nutritional Information (per serving):

Calories: 280, Carbs: 40g, Protein: 15g, Fat: 7g, Fiber: 6g

Avocado and Smoked Salmon Toast:

Preparation Time: 10 minutes

Serving: 1

Ingredients:

- 1 slice whole grain bread
- 1/2 ripe avocado
- 2 ounces smoked salmon
- Lemon juice and black pepper for seasoning

Instructions:

1. Toast the whole grain bread.
2. Mash the avocado and spread it on the toast.
3. Top with smoked salmon and season with lemon juice and black pepper.

Nutritional Information:

Calories: 320, Carbs: 20g, Protein: 18g, Fat: 20g, Fiber: 8g

Egg and Veggie Breakfast Burrito:

Cooking Time: 15 minutes

Serving: 1

Ingredients:

- 1 whole wheat tortilla
- 2 eggs (scrambled)
- Mixed vegetables (bell peppers, onions, spinach)
- Salsa for topping

Instructions:

1. Sauté mixed vegetables until tender.
2. Scramble eggs and add them to the vegetables.
3. Spoon the mixture onto a whole wheat tortilla and top with salsa.

Nutritional Information:

Calories: 290, Carbs: 25g, Protein: 18g, Fat: 12g, Fiber: 5g

Cottage Cheese and Berry Bowl:

Preparation Time: 5 minutes

Serving: 1

Ingredients:

- 1 cup low-fat cottage cheese
- Mixed berries (strawberries, blueberries, raspberries)
- 1 tablespoon flaxseeds (ground)

Instructions:

1. Combine cottage cheese with mixed berries.
2. Sprinkle with ground flaxseeds.

Nutritional Information:

Calories: 220, Carbs: 15g, Protein: 25g, Fat: 8g, Fiber: 6g

Sweet Potato and Spinach Frittata:

Cooking Time: 25 minutes

Serving: 4

Ingredients:

- 6 eggs
- 1 medium sweet potato (grated)
- Handful of fresh spinach
- 1/4 cup feta cheese (optional)

Instructions:

1. Preheat oven to 350°F (175°C).
2. Whisk eggs and fold in grated sweet potato, spinach, and feta.
3. Pour the mixture into a greased baking dish and bake until set.

Nutritional Information (per serving):

Calories: 180, Carbs: 10g, Protein: 12g, Fat: 10g, Fiber: 2g

Peanut Butter and Banana Smoothie:

Preparation Time: 5 minutes

Serving: 1

Ingredients:

- 1 banana
- 2 tablespoons peanut butter (unsweetened)
- 1/2 cup unsweetened almond milk
- Ice cubes (optional)

Instructions:

1. Blend banana, peanut butter, and almond milk until smooth.
2. Add ice cubes if desired and blend again.

Nutritional Information:

Calories: 280, Carbs: 30g, Protein: 8g, Fat: 15g, Fiber: 5g

Blueberry and Almond Overnight Oats:

Preparation Time: 10 minutes (plus overnight refrigeration)

Serving: 1

Ingredients:

- 1/2 cup rolled oats.
- 1/2 cup unsweetened almond milk
- 1/4 cup fresh blueberries
- 1 tablespoon almond slices

Instructions:

1. Combine rolled oats and almond milk in a jar; refrigerate overnight.
2. In the morning, top with fresh blueberries and almond slices.

Nutritional Information:

Calories: 280, Carbs: 40g, Protein: 8g, Fat: 10g, Fiber: 7g

Spinach and Feta Egg Muffins:

Cooking Time: 20 minutes

Serving: 2

Ingredients:

- 4 eggs
- 1 cup fresh spinach (chopped)
- 1/4 cup feta cheese (crumbled)
- Salt and pepper to taste

Instructions:

1. Preheat oven to 350°F (175°C).
2. In a bowl, whisk eggs and mix in spinach, feta, salt, and pepper.
3. Pour the mixture into greased muffin cups and bake until set.

Nutritional Information (per serving):

Calories: 180, Carbs: 2g, Protein: 14g, Fat: 12g, Fiber: 1g

Apple Cinnamon Chia Seed Pudding:

Preparation Time: 10 minutes (plus refrigeration time)

Serving: 1

Ingredients:

- 2 tablespoons chia seeds
- 1/2 cup unsweetened almond milk
- 1/2 apple (diced)
- 1/2 teaspoon cinnamon

Instructions:

1. Mix chia seeds and almond milk; refrigerate until a pudding-like consistency is achieved.
2. Layer with diced apples and sprinkle with cinnamon.

Nutritional Information:

Calories: 220, Carbs: 30g, Protein: 5g, Fat: 10g, Fiber: 10g

Turkey and Veggie Breakfast Wrap:

Cooking Time: 15 minutes

Serving: 1

Ingredients:

- 1 whole wheat tortilla
- 2 slices turkey bacon
- 1 egg (scrambled)
- Mixed vegetables (bell peppers, onions)

Instructions:

1. Cook turkey bacon and set aside.
2. Sauté mixed vegetables until tender, then add scrambled eggs.
3. Place the egg and veggie mixture on a whole wheat tortilla, top with turkey bacon, and fold into a wrap.

Nutritional Information:

Calories: 280, Carbs: 25g, Protein: 18g, Fat: 12g, Fiber: 5g

CHAPTER 4:

WHOLESOME LUNCH AND DINNER RECIPES

Grilled Chicken Salad with Quinoa:

Cooking Time: 30 minutes

Serving: 2

Ingredients:

- 2 boneless, skinless chicken breasts
- 1 cup cooked quinoa
- Mixed salad greens
- Cherry tomatoes, cucumber, and bell peppers
- Olive oil and balsamic vinegar for dressing

Instructions:

1. Grill chicken until fully cooked.
2. Assemble the salad with quinoa, mixed greens, and chopped vegetables.
3. Slice grilled chicken and place on top.
4. Drizzle with olive oil and balsamic vinegar.

Nutritional Information (per serving):

Calories: 350, Carbs: 30g, Protein: 30g, Fat: 12g, Fiber: 6g

Salmon and Vegetable Stir-Fry:

Cooking Time: 20 minutes

Serving: 2

Ingredients:

- 2 salmon fillets
- Mixed stir-fry vegetables (broccoli, bell peppers, snap peas)
- 2 tablespoons low-sodium soy sauce
- 1 tablespoon sesame oil
- 1 teaspoon grated ginger

Instructions:

1. Pan-sear salmon until cooked.
2. Stir-fry vegetables in sesame oil and ginger.
3. Add cooked salmon and soy sauce.

Nutritional Information (per serving):

Calories: 380, Carbs: 20g, Protein: 35g, Fat: 18g, Fiber: 7g

Vegetarian Chickpea and Spinach Curry:

Cooking Time: 25 minutes

Serving: 4

Ingredients:

- 1 can chickpeas (drained and rinsed)
- 2 cups fresh spinach
- 1 onion (chopped)
- 2 tomatoes (diced)
- 2 cloves garlic (minced)
- 1 tablespoon curry powder

Instructions:

1. Sauté onions and garlic until soft.
2. Add tomatoes, chickpeas, and curry powder, simmer.
3. Stir in fresh spinach until wilted.

Nutritional Information (per serving):

Calories: 280, Carbs: 45g, Protein: 12g, Fat: 6g, Fiber: 10g

Turkey and Quinoa Stuffed Peppers:

Cooking Time: 45 minutes

Serving: 4

Ingredients:

- 1 cup cooked quinoa
- 1 pound ground turkey
- 4 bell peppers (halved)
- 1 can black beans (drained)
- 1 cup diced tomatoes.
- Taco seasoning to taste

Instructions:

1. Brown turkey and season with taco seasoning.
2. Mix cooked quinoa, black beans, and diced tomatoes.
3. Stuff bell peppers with the mixture and bake until peppers are tender.

Nutritional Information (per serving):

Calories: 320, Carbs: 35g, Protein: 25g, Fat: 10g, Fiber: 8g

Mushroom and Spinach Stuffed Chicken Breast:

Cooking Time: 35 minutes

Serving: 2

Ingredients:

- 2 boneless, skinless chicken breasts
- 1 cup chopped mushrooms.
- 2 cups fresh spinach
- 2 cloves garlic (minced)
- 1 tablespoon olive oil

Instructions:

1. Sauté mushrooms and garlic in olive oil.
2. Add spinach until wilted.
3. Cut a pocket in each chicken breast and stuff with the mushroom-spinach mixture.
4. Bake until chicken is cooked through.

Nutritional Information (per serving):

Calories: 320, Carbs: 10g, Protein: 40g, Fat: 15g, Fiber: 4g

Lemon Garlic Shrimp with Zucchini Noodles:

Cooking Time: 20 minutes

Serving: 2

Ingredients:

- 1 pound shrimp (peeled and deveined)
- 2 zucchinis (spiralized into noodles)
- 2 tablespoons olive oil
- 2 cloves garlic (minced)
- Juice of 1 lemon

Instructions:

1. Sauté shrimp and garlic in olive oil until cooked.
2. Add zucchini noodles and cook until tender.
3. Squeeze lemon juice over the dish before serving.

Nutritional Information (per serving):

Calories: 250, Carbs: 10g, Protein: 30g, Fat: 12g, Fiber: 3g

Baked Cod with Roasted Vegetables:

Cooking Time: 30 minutes

Serving: 2

Ingredients:

- 2 cod fillets
- Assorted vegetables (carrots, Brussels sprouts, cherry tomatoes)
- 2 tablespoons olive oil
- Fresh herbs (rosemary, thyme)

Instructions:

1. Season cod with herbs and bake until flaky.
2. Toss vegetables in olive oil and roast until tender.
3. Serve cod on a bed of roasted vegetables.

Nutritional Information (per serving):

Calories: 280, Carbs: 20g, Protein: 30g, Fat: 12g, Fiber: 8g

Cauliflower Fried Rice with Tofu:

Cooking Time: 25 minutes

Serving: 4

Ingredients:

- 1 head cauliflower (riced)
- 1 cup tofu (cubed)
- Mixed vegetables (peas, carrots, green onions)
- 2 eggs (scrambled)
- Low-sodium soy sauce to taste

Instructions:

1. Sauté tofu until golden.
2. Add mixed vegetables and cauliflower rice; cook until vegetables are tender.
3. Stir in scrambled eggs and soy sauce.

Nutritional Information (per serving):

Calories: 220, Carbs: 20g, Protein: 15g, Fat: 10g, Fiber: 8g

Lentil and Vegetable Stew:

Cooking Time: 40 minutes

Serving: 4

Ingredients:

- 1 cup dry lentils (rinsed)
- 2 carrots (diced)
- 2 celery stalks (chopped)
- 1 onion (chopped)
- 3 cloves garlic (minced)
- 4 cups vegetable broth

Instructions:

1. Sauté onions and garlic until softened.
2. Add lentils, carrots, celery, and vegetable broth; simmer until lentils are tender.
3. Season to taste with herbs and spices.

Nutritional Information (per serving):

Calories: 280, Carbs: 45g, Protein: 18g, Fat: 2g, Fiber: 15g

Sweet Potato and Black Bean Chili:

Cooking Time: 30 minutes

Serving: 4

Ingredients:

- 2 sweet potatoes (cubed)
- 1 can black beans (drained and rinsed)
- 1 can diced tomatoes
- 1 onion (chopped)
- Chili powder and cumin to taste

Instructions:

1. Sauté onions until translucent.
2. Add sweet potatoes, black beans, diced tomatoes, and spices.
3. Simmer until sweet potatoes are tender.

Nutritional Information (per serving):

Calories: 320, Carbs: 60g, Protein: 15g, Fat: 2g, Fiber: 12g

Chicken and Broccoli Quinoa Bowl:

Cooking Time: 25 minutes

Serving: 2

Ingredients:

- 2 boneless, skinless chicken breasts
- 1 cup quinoa (cooked)
- Broccoli florets
- 2 tablespoons low-sodium soy sauce
- 1 tablespoon honey

Instructions:

1. Grill or bake chicken until fully cooked.
2. Steam broccoli until tender.
3. Mix quinoa, chicken, and broccoli.
4. Drizzle with a sauce made from soy sauce and honey.

Nutritional Information (per serving):

Calories: 350, Carbs: 45g, Protein: 30g, Fat: 8g, Fiber: 6g

Mediterranean Chickpea Salad:

Preparation Time: 15 minutes

Serving: 4

Ingredients:

- 2 cans chickpeas (drained and rinsed)
- Cherry tomatoes (halved)
- Cucumber (diced)
- Kalamata olives
- Feta cheese (crumbled)
- Olive oil and lemon juice for dressing

Instructions:

1. Combine chickpeas, cherry tomatoes, cucumber, olives, and feta in a bowl.
2. Drizzle with olive oil and lemon juice; toss to coat.

Nutritional Information (per serving):

Calories: 280, Carbs: 40g, Protein: 15g, Fat: 10g, Fiber: 12g

Turkey and Vegetable Skewers with Quinoa:

Cooking Time: 20 minutes

Serving: 2

Ingredients:

- 1 pound turkey breast (cut into cubes)
- Assorted vegetables (bell peppers, cherry tomatoes, zucchini)
- 1 cup quinoa (cooked)
- Olive oil and herbs for marinating

Instructions:

1. Marinate turkey cubes in olive oil and herbs.
2. Thread turkey and vegetables onto skewers and grill until turkey is cooked.
3. Serve over a bed of cooked quinoa.

Nutritional Information (per serving):

Calories: 320, Carbs: 30g, Protein: 35g, Fat: 8g, Fiber: 6g

Eggplant and Chickpea Stew:

Cooking Time: 35 minutes

Serving: 4

Ingredients:

- 1 large eggplant (cubed)
- 1 can chickpeas (drained and rinsed)
- 2 tomatoes (diced)
- 1 onion (chopped)
- 3 cloves garlic (minced)
- Vegetable broth and spices to taste

Instructions:

1. Sauté onions and garlic until softened.
2. Add eggplant, chickpeas, tomatoes, and vegetable broth; simmer until eggplant is tender.
3. Season with your choice of spices.

Nutritional Information (per serving):

Calories: 250, Carbs: 40g, Protein: 10g, Fat: 5g, Fiber: 12g

Tofu and Vegetable Stir-Fry with Brown Rice:

Cooking Time: 30 minutes

Serving: 4

Ingredients:

- 1 block firm tofu (pressed and cubed)
- Mixed stir-fry vegetables (broccoli, snap peas, carrots)
- 2 cups cooked brown rice
- Low-sodium soy sauce and ginger for flavoring

Instructions:

1. Sauté tofu until golden and set aside.
2. Stir-fry mixed vegetables until tender.
3. Add tofu back into the pan and season with soy sauce and ginger.
4. Serve over a bed of cooked brown rice.

Nutritional Information (per serving):

Calories: 320, Carbs: 50g, Protein: 15g, Fat: 8g, Fiber: 8g

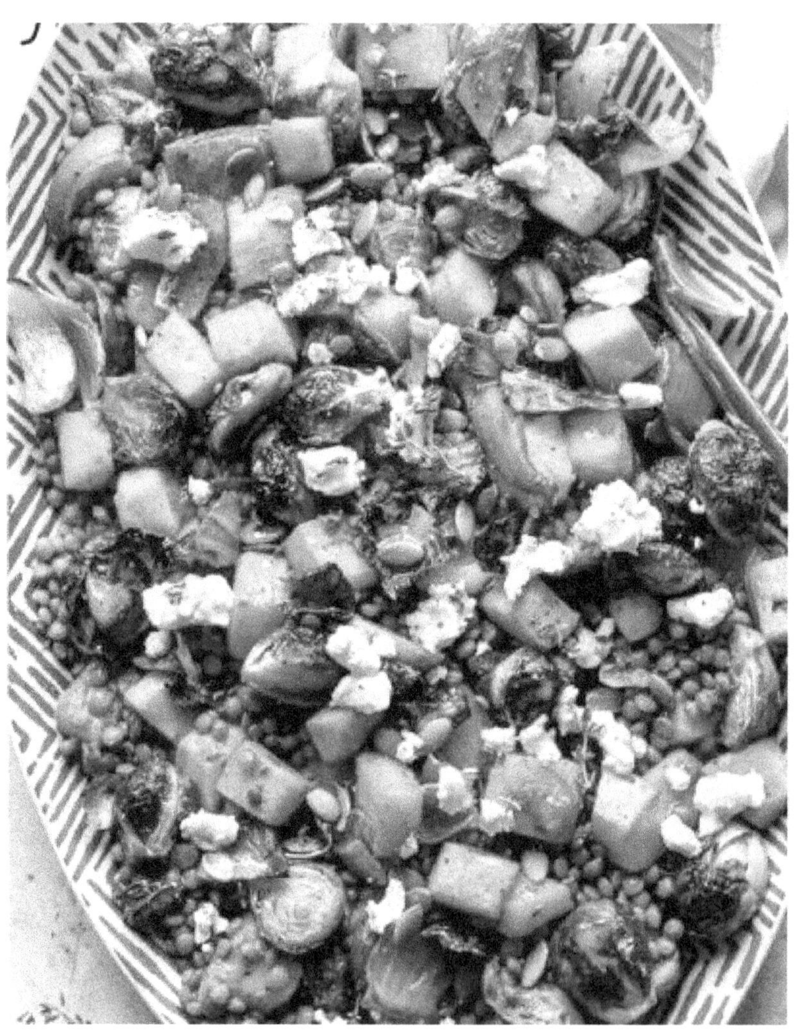

CHAPTER 5

SNACKS AND TREATS FOR PCOS AND

DIABETES

Greek Yogurt and Berry Parfait:

Preparation Time: 5 minutes

Serving: 1

Ingredients:

- 1 cup Greek yogurt
- Mixed berries (strawberries, blueberries)
- 1 tablespoon chia seeds

Instructions:

1. Layer Greek yogurt with mixed berries in a glass.
2. Top with chia seeds.

Nutritional Information:

Calories: 200, Carbs: 25g, Protein: 15g, Fat: 7g, Fiber: 6g

Cucumber and Hummus Bites:

Preparation Time: 10 minutes

Serving: 1

Ingredients:

- Cucumber slices
- Hummus
- Cherry tomatoes (halved)

Instructions:

1. Spread hummus on cucumber slices.
2. Top with halved cherry tomatoes.

Nutritional Information:

Calories: 120, Carbs: 15g, Protein: 5g, Fat: 6g, Fiber: 5g

Almond and Dark Chocolate Energy Bites:

Preparation Time: 15 minutes

Serving: 2

Ingredients:

- 1/2 cup almonds (chopped)
- 1/4 cup dark chocolate chips
- 2 tablespoons almond butter
- 1 tablespoon honey

Instructions:

1. Mix almonds, dark chocolate chips, almond butter, and honey.
2. Form into bite-sized balls.

Nutritional Information (per serving):

Calories: 180, Carbs: 15g, Protein: 5g, Fat: 12g, Fiber: 3g

Yogurt and Almond Berry Popsicles:

Preparation Time: 10 minutes (plus freezing time)

Serving: 4

Ingredients:

- 2 cups Greek yogurt
- Mixed berries (raspberries, blueberries)
- 1/4 cup almonds (chopped)

Instructions:

1. Mix Greek yogurt, mixed berries, and chopped almonds.
2. Pour into popsicle molds and freeze.

Nutritional Information (per serving):

Calories: 120, Carbs: 15g, Protein: 8g, Fat: 4g, Fiber: 3g

Avocado and Tomato Salsa with Whole Grain Crackers:

Preparation Time: 15 minutes

Serving: 2

Ingredients:

- 1 avocado (diced)
- 1 cup cherry tomatoes (diced)
- Red onion (finely chopped)
- Cilantro (chopped)
- Whole grain crackers

Instructions:

1. Mix diced avocado, tomatoes, red onion, and cilantro.
2. Serve with whole grain crackers.

Nutritional Information (per serving):

Calories: 160, Carbs: 20g, Protein: 4g, Fat: 9g, Fiber: 6g

Cottage Cheese and Pineapple Bowl:

Preparation Time: 5 minutes

Serving: 1

Ingredients:

- 1/2 cup low-fat cottage cheese
- Fresh pineapple chunks
- 1 tablespoon flaxseeds (ground)

Instructions:

1. Combine cottage cheese with fresh pineapple.
2. Sprinkle with ground flaxseeds.

Nutritional Information:

Calories: 150, Carbs: 20g, Protein: 12g, Fat: 4g, Fiber: 3g

Baked Sweet Potato Fries with Greek Yogurt Dip:

Preparation Time: 30 minutes

Serving: 2

Ingredients:

- 2 sweet potatoes (cut into fries)
- 1 tablespoon olive oil
- 1 teaspoon paprika
- 1 cup Greek yogurt
- Fresh dill (chopped)

Instructions:

1. Toss sweet potato fries with olive oil and paprika.
2. Bake until crispy.
3. Mix Greek yogurt with chopped dill for dipping.

Nutritional Information (per serving):

Calories: 180, Carbs: 25g, Protein: 10g, Fat: 5g, Fiber: 4g

Chia Seed Pudding with Berries:

Preparation Time: 5 minutes (plus refrigeration time)

Serving: 1

Ingredients:

- 2 tablespoons chia seeds
- 1/2 cup unsweetened almond milk
- Mixed berries (strawberries, blueberries)

Instructions:

1. Mix chia seeds and almond milk; refrigerate until a pudding-like consistency is achieved.
2. Top with mixed berries.

Nutritional Information:

Calories: 160, Carbs: 20g, Protein: 5g, Fat: 8g, Fiber: 8g

Rice Cake with Peanut Butter and Banana:

Preparation Time: 5 minutes

Serving: 1

Ingredients:

- 1 rice cake
- 1 tablespoon natural peanut butter
- 1/2 banana (sliced)

Instructions:

1. Spread peanut butter on a rice cake.
2. Top with sliced banana.

Nutritional Information:

Calories: 180, Carbs: 20g, Protein: 6g, Fat: 9g, Fiber: 3g

Caprese Skewers with Balsamic Glaze:

Preparation Time: 10 minutes

Serving: 2

Ingredients:

- Cherry tomatoes
- Mozzarella balls
- Fresh basil leaves
- Balsamic glaze

Instructions:

1. Thread cherry tomatoes, mozzarella balls, and basil leaves onto skewers.
2. Drizzle with balsamic glaze before serving.

Nutritional Information (per serving):

Calories: 160, Carbs: 10g, Protein: 8g, Fat: 10g, Fiber: 2g

Apple and Almond Butter Sandwiches:

Preparation Time: 5 minutes

Serving: 1

Ingredients:

- 1 apple (sliced)
- Natural almond butter
- Granola (optional)

Instructions:

1. Spread almond butter on apple slices.
2. Create sandwiches and sprinkle with granola if desired.

Nutritional Information:

Calories: 200, Carbs: 25g, Protein: 4g, Fat: 10g, Fiber: 5g

Roasted Chickpeas with Cumin and Paprika:

Preparation Time: 30 minutes

Serving: 4

Ingredients:

- 2 cans chickpeas (drained and rinsed)
- 1 tablespoon olive oil
- 1 teaspoon cumin
- 1 teaspoon paprika

Instructions:

1. Toss chickpeas in olive oil, cumin, and paprika.
2. Roast until crispy.

Nutritional Information (per serving):

Calories: 160, Carbs: 25g, Protein: 7g, Fat: 5g, Fiber: 6g

Chocolate Avocado Mousse:

Preparation Time: 10 minutes

Serving: 2

Ingredients:

- 2 ripe avocados
- 1/4 cup cocoa powder
- 1/4 cup honey or maple syrup
- 1 teaspoon vanilla extract

Instructions:

1. Blend avocados, cocoa powder, honey (or maple syrup), and vanilla extract until smooth.
2. Chill before serving.

Nutritional Information (per serving):

Calories: 250, Carbs: 30g, Protein: 4g, Fat: 15g, Fiber: 8g

Turkey and Cheese Lettuce Wraps:

Preparation Time: 10 minutes

Serving: 2

Ingredients:

- Deli turkey slices
- Cheese slices
- Lettuce leaves
- Mustard or low-fat dressing

Instructions:

1. Layer turkey and cheese on lettuce leaves.
2. Roll and secure with toothpicks.
3. Serve with mustard or a low-fat dressing for dipping.

Nutritional Information (per serving):

Calories: 180, Carbs: 3g, Protein: 20g, Fat: 10g, Fiber: 1g

Homemade Trail Mix:

Preparation Time: 5 minutes

Serving: 4

Ingredients:

- Almonds
- Walnuts
- Pumpkin seeds
- Dried cranberries
- Dark chocolate chips

Instructions:

1. Mix almonds, walnuts, pumpkin seeds, dried cranberries, and dark chocolate chips in a bowl.
2. Portion into small snack bags.

Nutritional Information (per serving):

Calories: 200, Carbs: 15g, Protein: 6g, Fat: 15g, Fiber: 4g

CHAPTER 6

14-DAY MEAL PLAN

Day 1:

- Breakfast: Blueberry and Almond Overnight Oats
- Lunch: Grilled Chicken Salad with Quinoa
- Dinner: Lentil and Vegetable Stew

Day 2:

- Breakfast: Spinach and Feta Egg Muffins
- Lunch: Turkey and Quinoa Stuffed Peppers
- Dinner: Baked Cod with Roasted Vegetables

Day 3:

- Breakfast: Apple Cinnamon Chia Seed Pudding
- Lunch: Mediterranean Chickpea Salad
- Dinner: Chicken and Broccoli Quinoa Bowl

Day 4:

- Breakfast: Peanut Butter and Banana Smoothie
- Lunch: Sweet Potato and Black Bean Chili
- Dinner: Tofu and Vegetable Stir-Fry with Brown Rice

Day 5:

- Breakfast: Blueberry and Almond Overnight Oats
- Lunch: Turkey and Veggie Breakfast Wrap
- Dinner: Eggplant and Chickpea Stew

Day 6:

- Breakfast: Mango and Kale Smoothie Bowl
- Lunch: Lentil and Vegetable Stew
- Dinner: Cauliflower Fried Rice with Tofu

Day 7:

- Breakfast: Spinach and Feta Egg Muffins
- Lunch: Mushroom and Spinach Stuffed Chicken Breast
- Dinner: Roasted Chickpeas with Cumin and Paprika

Day 8:

- Breakfast: Blueberry and Almond Overnight Oats
- Lunch: Turkey and Quinoa Stuffed Peppers
- Dinner: Baked Cod with Roasted Vegetables

Day 9:

- Breakfast: Peanut Butter and Banana Smoothie
- Lunch: Mediterranean Chickpea Salad
- Dinner: Tofu and Vegetable Stir-Fry with Brown Rice

Day 10:

- Breakfast: Apple Cinnamon Chia Seed Pudding
- Lunch: Sweet Potato and Black Bean Chili
- Dinner: Lentil and Vegetable Stew

Day 11:

- Breakfast: Blueberry and Almond Overnight Oats
- Lunch: Turkey and Veggie Breakfast Wrap
- Dinner: Eggplant and Chickpea Stew

Day 12:

- Breakfast: Mango and Kale Smoothie Bowl
- Lunch: Chicken and Broccoli Quinoa Bowl
- Dinner: Cauliflower Fried Rice with Tofu

Day 13:

- Breakfast: Greek Yogurt and Berry Parfait
- Lunch: Turkey and Cheese Lettuce Wraps
- Dinner: Homemade Trail Mix

Day 14:

- Breakfast: Chia Seed Pudding with Berries
- Lunch: Caprese Skewers with Balsamic Glaze
- Dinner: Chocolate Avocado Mousse

CONCLUSION

As we draw the curtains on this culinary journey through the pages of "Harmony in Every Bite," I am reminded of the countless lives touched by the power of mindful nutrition. From the initial spark of hope that ignited within Sophie to the potential for transformation within you, dear reader, this cookbook transcends the boundaries of a mere collection of recipes.

The stories within these pages are not just narratives of health and wellness; they are tales of resilience, triumph, and the indomitable spirit of those facing the challenges of PCOS and diabetes. Through the alchemy of flavors and the careful orchestration of nutrients, we have crafted a symphony that resonates with the promise of a brighter, healthier future.

As you delve into these recipes, I invite you to savor not only the flavors but also the emotions woven into each dish. It is my sincere hope that this cookbook becomes a companion on your journey to well-being, a source of inspiration during moments of doubt, and a guiding light when the path ahead seems obscured.

Your feedback is invaluable to me. The heart and soul poured into these recipes are a reflection of my commitment to helping you navigate the complexities of PCOS and diabetes. I invite you to share your experiences, your triumphs, and even your challenges. Your insights will not only contribute to the refinement of these recipes but will also create a supportive community bound by a common goal – a life of harmony and health.

Every comment, suggestion, and shared story becomes a building block in the foundation of a community united by a shared journey. Together, we can turn the tide against the challenges posed by PCOS and diabetes, celebrating the victories, both big and small, that come with each carefully crafted meal.

Thank you for entrusting me with a part of your health journey. May the recipes within these pages continue to serve as a source of nourishment, both for your body and your spirit. Here's to a future filled with health, harmony, and the joy found in every bite.

With gratitude and warmest wishes.

BONUS:

PCOS AND DIABETES-FRIENDLY

GROCERY SHOPPING

Managing both PCOS (Polycystic Ovary Syndrome) and diabetes involves making mindful choices when it comes to grocery shopping. Here are some tips to help you make nutritious and balanced selections:

Shopping for Fresh Produce:

Prioritize Colorful Vegetables: Opt for a variety of colorful vegetables such as leafy greens, bell peppers, broccoli, and carrots. These are rich in vitamins, minerals, and antioxidants.

Include Low-Glycemic Fruits: Choose fruits with a lower glycemic index, such as berries, cherries, and apples. These fruits have a milder impact on blood sugar levels.

Incorporate Fresh Herbs: Add flavor to your meals with fresh herbs like basil, cilantro, and parsley. They provide taste without added sugars or unhealthy fats.

Choosing Lean Proteins:

Select Lean Meats: Choose lean protein sources like skinless poultry, turkey, lean cuts of beef or pork, and fish. These options are lower in saturated fats.

Include Plant-Based Proteins: Incorporate plant-based protein sources such as tofu, tempeh, legumes, and lentils. These can be excellent alternatives to animal proteins.

Opt for Skinless Poultry: If you enjoy poultry, choose skinless options to reduce saturated fat intake.

Smart Carbohydrate Choices:

Prioritize Whole Grains: Opt for whole grains like brown rice, quinoa, oats, and whole wheat bread over refined grains. Whole grains provide more fiber and nutrients.

Control Portion Sizes: Be mindful of portion sizes when consuming carbohydrates. This can help regulate blood sugar levels and manage weight.

Choose Legumes: Incorporate legumes like beans and lentils into your meals. They are rich in fiber and protein, which can aid in blood sugar control.

Healthy Fats for PCOS and Diabetes:

Embrace Heart-Healthy Oils: Use heart-healthy oils like olive oil, avocado oil, and canola oil for cooking. These oils are rich in monounsaturated fats.

Include Omega-3 Fatty Acids: Incorporate sources of omega-3 fatty acids, such as fatty fish (salmon, mackerel) and flaxseeds. These fats have anti-inflammatory properties.

Limit Saturated and Trans Fats: Reduce intake of saturated and trans fats found in fried foods, processed snacks, and certain baked goods. These fats can contribute to inflammation and insulin resistance.

Additional Tips:

Read Nutrition Labels: Familiarize yourself with nutrition labels to make informed choices about the products you buy. Look for lower sugar and whole, unprocessed ingredients.

Stay Hydrated: Water is essential for overall health. Choose water or herbal teas over sugary beverages to stay hydrated.

Plan Your Meals: Plan your meals and snacks in advance to ensure a well-balanced diet. This can help you make healthier choices and avoid impulsive purchases.